BURSITIS CURE

A Definitive step by step guide on the best treatment for Bursitis

By

Dr. Harvey Donald

Copyright @ 2024

Table of Contents

PREFACE

This book will definitely guide you on what you ought to know and fully understand about Bursitis and its treatment options. The manual will guide you on the signs and symptoms of bursitis, types of bursitis, causes and risk factors of bursitis, diagnostic tests for bursitis, prevention and treatment options, bursitis surgery and so much more.

CHAPTER ONE

INTRODUCTION

Bursitis is an inflammation (irritation) of the bursae or a throbbing condition that affects the small, fluid-filled sacs referred to as **Bursae.** The Bursae which are more than 150 in the human body are fluid-filled sacs located around your joints that surrounds, lubricates, or shields the areas where tendons, skin, and muscle tissues meet bones.

Inflamed bursae which results into pain and discomfort in the affected location limit the ways an individual can move their joints.

Injury, excessive-use, or inflammation from gout or an autoimmune condition such as *rheumatoid arthritis* may result into bursitis.

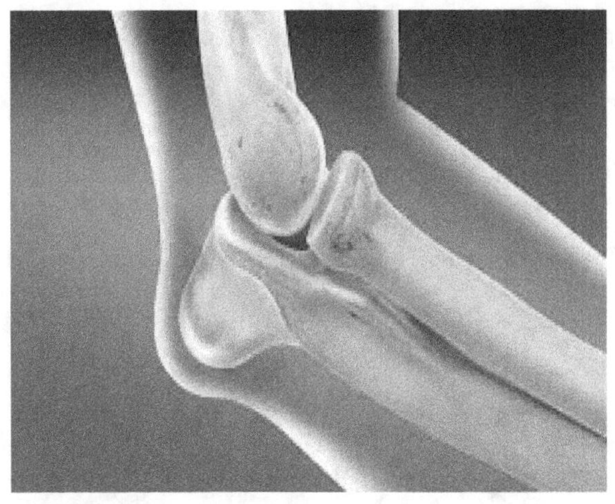

The elbow, hip, and shoulder, knee, heel and at the base of your large or big toe are all common locations for bursitis. Bursitis usually occurs close to the joints that perform regular repetitive motion with treatment generally involving resting the affected joint and cushioning it from excessive trauma. Bursitis can also be prevented by taking breaks during recurrent tasks and warming up before exercise.

CHAPTER TWO

BURSITIS AND ITS TYPES

Bursitis can occur quickly, or it can be ongoing (chronic), although when it comes on abruptly, it often hurts to move your affected joint. With chronic bursitis, there is a gradually swelling of the bursa which may result into you feeling pain or sometimes not feeling any pain at all.

Oftentimes, bursitis is caused by an infection and this is referred to as ***septic bursitis.*** Despite the fact that septic bursitis is somewhat uncommon, it is important for your physician to check in order to ensure you don't have an infection.

Some common types of bursitis may include:

(a) **ELBOW BURSITIS-** One of the most common locations of bursitis is at the pointy part of your elbow and thus, if you have elbow bursitis (olecranon bursitis), the bottom of your elbow will be swollen, red, and painful, with pain that gets aggravated when you tend to bend it. As a result of the swelling, it can appear like that there is a small ball beneath your skin. Nevertheless, if the ball gets larger, it can make it difficult to move your elbow.

Leaning on your elbows excessively can result into elbow bursitis. Electricians, plumbers, HVAC (heating, ventilation, and air conditioning) technicians, and other individuals who have to crawl into tight spaces for work are more probably to exert pressure on their elbows as they perform their jobs or tasks.

Bumps or injuries can also result into elbow bursitis. Physicians don't ascertain why, but individuals who get dialysis for kidney issues are more probably to get elbow bursitis.

Furthermore, to help relieve your pain, an elastic bandage should be wrapped around your elbow or you can just wear elbow pads. If you perform work or tasks that exert pressure on your elbows, wearing elbow pads or making use of a padded mat can help in preventing bursitis.

(b) **Shoulder Bursitis-** Shoulder bursitis (subacromial bursitis) results into painful swelling in your shoulder that gets aggravated specifically when you move it. This can be as a result of an injury or a bump. Some individual's shoulder bones are basically shaped in a manner that puts extra pressure on the bursa. You are more probably to get shoulder bursitis if your bones are shaped like this.

Depending on how awful the swelling is, you might not have the ability of moving your shoulder, a condition referred to as ***frozen shoulder or adhesive capsulitis.*** Consult your physician if it hurts too much to move your shoulder. Your physician can perform tests to check if it is bursitis or a different condition. Furthermore, your physician may recommend physical therapy for your shoulder or other form of treatment therapies.

(c) **Hip Bursitis-** One common location of bursitis is at the bony part of your hip that bulges out close to your waist. You might experience pain in your hip or outer thigh if you have this kind of bursitis.

You might not observe any swelling if you have bursitis in your hip, although it can be painful. Initially, the pain usually feels sharp, and then turns into an ache that extends across your hip. It might ache more when you lay on your hip, hunch, walk up the stairs, or stand up from sitting down.

You are more probably to get hip bursitis if you have issues with your back or hips, if you were born with one leg that is somewhat shorter than the other leg or if you have ever had a hip replacement surgery (hip arthroplasty). Exercises like riding a bike, running, or climbing up or walking up a stairs can inflame it. You have a higher risk of getting hip bursitis if you have a job where you have to stand up for extended periods (*such as being a cashier, a server, or a warehouse worker*) or where you have to move things that are extremely heavy.

Your physician might tell you to walk with a cane or make use of crutches if you have hip bursitis (**trochanteric or iliopectineal bursitis**). This therapy will make the hip bursitis heal quicker. Your physician might watch you sit, and stand, walk, or even videotape you as this will aid your physician in teaching you less painful ways of standing or moving around.

(d) **KNEE BURSITIS-** There are numerous several parts of your knee that can get bursitis, such as *close to your kneecap (prepatellar bursitis) or on the inside of your knee* and if your bursitis is in your kneecap, it is more likely to be as a result of an infection.

When you develop or have bursitis, it usually hurts to move or exert pressure on your knee, and it can ache if another individual touches it. Your knee might also feel warmer than the other parts of your body, and it oftentimes appears red or swollen.

Oftentimes, knee bursitis comes on quickly after an injury or bump to knee. Occasionally, it is as a result of pressure to your knee joints over the years and the pain comes on gradually.

If you engage in these kinds of work, you should make use of a padded cushion or board beneath your knee and take as much breaks as you can. Knee pads can also be worn, although try not to squat or hunch for extended period of time. Stretching your hamstrings and other muscles prior to exercise can help in avoiding knee bursitis.

Individuals who fall a lot, like *wrestlers* and individuals who play sports *such as football* are more likely to get knee bursitis since they are more likely to fall on their knees or to bump.

Your physician will check both your knees, even if only one knee aches, to compare them to each other and ascertain what is wrong. Your physician might suggest you wear a wrap or knee brace as this will stimulate faster healing as well as protect your knees subsequently. Placing your knee up on a pillow can help in reducing the swelling.

(e) **FOOT BURSITIS-** There are around 33 joints in your feet, and most of the joints have bursa sacs to shield or protect them. Bursitis can be developed around your feet if any of these bursa sacs get inflamed. Around your Achilles tendon in the back of your foot, at the base of your toes, in between the outside of your small toe and your ankle or close to your heel are all common locations where bursitis can be developed.

Your foot might feel stiff, swollen or even painful if you have foot bursitis. The pain might get aggravated when you run, walk, or stand on your tip-toes.

High heels and shoes that compress your feet or don't fit you appropriately can result into bursitis. Dancers, runners as well as athletes are more likely to develop or get foot bursitis.

You can prevent foot bursitis by wearing supportive shoes that fit you appropriately as well as stretching your feet and legs prior to exercise.

Your physician might suggest you consult a podiatrist if you have foot bursitis. A physician who treats or takes care of feet and ankles is a **podiatrist** and since they are specialized in that field, the podiatrist might offer you a plastic or piece of foam referred to as an *orthotic* to put in your shoe in order to lubricate or cushion the foot.

(f) **BUTTOCKS BURSITIS-** Buttock bursitis (ischial bursitis) is when a bursa close to the main muscle of your buttocks becomes irritated and this type of bursitis is oftentimes referred to as *"weaver's bottom"* or *"tailor's bottom"* since it is more common in individuals who usually sit on hard surfaces, like the floor or chairs that are not padded.

This type of bursitis can result into pain and aching in your buttocks and around your thighs with the pain often aggravated after you sit for an extended period of time, stretch or after an exercise. It might also ache when you extend, flex or move your hips.

To make sitting more comfortable, you can make use of a donut-shaped pillow and also making use of a cold compress on the area can help you feel better.

CHAPTER THREE

SYMPTOMS AND SIGNS OF BURSITIS

Bursitis is most likely felt when you stretch or extend the joint, and you may have a restricted range of motion or movement even without pain.

Symptoms can also include:

(a) Joint stiffness

(b) Redness around the joint

(c) Joint swelling

(d) Skin redness or *erythema* which can appear somewhat darker on dark skin tones.

(e) Bursae thickening

(f) Hotness around the affected area

Types of bursitis and their associated symptoms

1. **Knee bursitis (prepatellar bursitis)**

- Difficulty in bending the leg.

2. **Foot bursitis (rectrocalcaneal bursitis)**

   - Difficulty in walking

3. **Elbow bursitis (olecranon bursitis)**

   - Difficulty in bending your arm

4. **Hip bursitis (Trochanteric bursitis)**

   - Pain particularly when you lie on your hip.

It is recommended you consult your physician if you experience:

(a) Debilitating joint pain that prevents movement.

(b) Trouble in moving a joint as well as a sharp or shooting pain particularly when you exercise yourself.

(c) Excessive redness, swelling, bruising or warmth around the affected area.

(d) A fever of over 102°F

(e) Pain that lasts longer than 14 days as well as a general illness.

CHAPTER FOUR

CAUSES AND RISK FACTORS OF BURSITIS

The most prevalent causes of bursitis are damage to your bursae or an injury to your bursae. The damage may bring about pain, redness as well as swelling in the affected area, although caused tend to be different for each type of bursitis.

Types of Bursitis and their causes

1. **ELBOW BURSITIS (Olecranon bursitis)**

   Causes
   - Frequently resting your elbows on hard surfaces or a hard blow to the back of the elbow.
   - Infection or a *gout*

Gout which can result in tophi or small nodules and can be felt within the bursa occurs when uric acid crystals accumulate in the body.

2. KNEE BURSITIS (Prepatellar bursitis)

Causes

- Infection and sports-related activities.
- Staying on your knees for extended periods of time
- Bending on your knees continually
- Sports-associated activities

Damage or tears to your knee bursae or kneecaps (patella) may result into swelling.

3. FOOT BURSITIS (Retrocalcaneal bursitis)

Causes

- Jumping, running or other frequent (repetitive) activities for an extended period of time.
- Starting a vigorous exercise without adequately warming up.
- Wearing shoes that are extremely tight at the back of the heel can aggravate since it rubs against the bursae.

4. HIP BURSITIS (Trochanteric bursitis)

Causes

- Injury and any condition that affects your bones like *arthritis*.
- Irregular posture while standing or sitting.

Other classifications of bursitis include the septic or infectious bursitis and the aseptic or noninfectious bursitis.

The septic or infectious bursitis typically occurs when the bursa becomes swollen or inflamed as a result of an infection from bacteria. This often takes place when bacteria are directly introduced into the bursa via a wound in the surrounding skin.

Septic bursitis can be caused by skin infections like cellulitis and also blood or joint infections which can also spread to the bursa. Septic bursitis which results in chills, fever, and other symptoms of infection causes the bursa to become red, hot, inflamed, or swollen.

Aseptic or noninfectious bursitis which have similar symptom to the septic bursitis is often caused by constant minor trauma to the joint area or strain injury.

Risk factors associated with bursitis

(a) Awkward posture

(b) Aging as well as injuries to the bursae

(c) Taking part or participating in repetitive sports as well as repetitive use of a given joint.

(d) Having a chronic medical condition and also getting an infection that can easily spread to your bones, joints, or bursae.

(e) Certain health conditions such as *rheumatoid arthritis, gout, and scleroderma* can cause bursitis.

CHAPTER FIVE

DIAGNOSTIC TESTS FOR BURSITIS

Bursitis can usually be diagnosed by physical examination and medical history, although other tests can also be used in diagnosing bursitis and also to rule out the possibility of a more severe condition.

An individual can also be asked about any recent activities that may be causing joint stress.

Your physician can make use of an X-ray to diagnose bursitis as they help to exclude other causes of your discomfort as well as check for broken or fractured bones. Furthermore, if your bursitis can't be easily diagnosed by a physical examination alone, ultrasound or MRI (magnetic resonance imaging scan) might be used to check for possible tendon or joint damage.

If you have a high temperature, your physician can take small fluid samples from the affected bursae. Your healthcare professional might order blood tests or an analysis of fluid from the swollen bursa to identify the cause of Joint pain and swelling. Blood tests helps in assessing for rheumatoid arthritis.

Needle aspiration is regularly suggested in instances where infectious bursitis seems to be limited to the joint. In some instances, such as when an individual has **elbow bursitis (olecranon bursitis),** carrying out a needle aspiration will elevate the risk of a secondary infection moving from the skin into the bursa.

Empiric therapy which involves administering antibiotics before clinical observation can also be performed.

CHAPTER SIX

PREVENTION AND TREATMENT OF BURSITIS

Bursitis is not often preventable, although making some fundamental lifestyle changes can decrease your risk of developing bursitis as well as preventing intense flare-ups.

Bursitis can be prevented by:

(a) Maintaining a healthy body weight to prevent putting additional pressure on the joints.

(b) Taking regular breaks when carrying out repetitive tasks or other activities.

(c) Bending your knees when you lift. Failing to do so exerts additional stress on the bursae in your hips.

(d) Making use of a dolly or wheeled cart while carrying heavy loads. Carrying or wheeling heavy loads puts stress on the bursae in your shoulders.

(e) Exercising to enhance the muscles supporting the joints as well as to help protect the affected joint

(f) Stretching and warming up before beginning arduous activities. This will help in protecting the joints from any form of injury.

(g) Making use of kneeling pads to decrease the pressure on your knees if your hobby or job requires much kneeling.

(h) Discontinuing an activity if you experience pain sensation.

(i) Inserting an orthotic shoe to help in decreasing the risk of hip bursitis as well as preventing hip bursitis.

(j) Practicing excellent posture when sitting as well as standing.

(k) Avoiding smoking tobacco.

Bursitis typically gets better on its own, nevertheless conservative measures such as rest, icing the joint, and pain medication may alleviate your bursitis.

Other treatment options for bursitis:

(a) **Corticosteroids-** Corticosteroids can be used in mitigating pain, swelling, and inflammation in as much there is no proof of any infection in or around the bursa. Use of corticosteroids typically works instantly and, in many instances, one injection is all you require.

(b) **Use of antibiotics-** Antibiotics are vital in cases in which the bursa is infected.

(c) **Use of assisitive device-** Temporary use of a walking cane or other devices such as *crutches* *or brace, split or elastic bandage* will help in mitigating pressure on the affected area.

(d) **Home exercises-** At-home exercises may help in alleviating pain and other symptoms, although in rare cases, physical therapy is required. Physical therapy can help in strengthening the muscles in the affected area to relieve pain and prevent recurrence.

SURGERY

Surgical procedure to remove a bursa within a joint when it becomes inflamed is referred to as **bursectomy.**

A bursectomy is a somewhat simple and invasive technique that is generally done arthroscopically on an outpatient basis. In this procedure, the bursa is removed via a small incision with a tiny camera. Since the surgery is much less invasive, recovery is faster and less painful.

A restricted or limited range of motion in a joint as a result of bursitis or other associated conditions may give rise to a recommendation for a bursectomy surgery. A primary aim of a bursectomy surgery is to mitigate the physical impairments caused by swollen, inflamed or enlarged bursae.

Rest, physical therapy and medications which often resolve most problem conditions are the most common treatment for bursitis, although these approaches no longer treat symptoms effectively, a bursectomy surgery may be your ideal option for sustained relief.

Benefits of Bursectomy surgery

There are numerous unique benefits to a bursectomy surgery and some of the benefits include:

(a) **Quick pain relief-** One of the main benefits of a bursectomy surgery is the potential for substantial relief of symptoms, most particularly *pain.* By getting rid of or removing the inflamed bursa, the source of pain is directly addressed, thus allowing individuals to experience instant relief.

(b) **Improved quality of life-** A bursectomy surgery can contribute to an enhanced overall quality of life which includes *daily tasks around the house, ability to achieve or accomplish work effectively as well as more physical recreation activities.*

(c) **Improved Joint mobility-** This technique aims to enhance joint mobility, thus allowing patients to take part in more activities than they were initially able.

(d) Prevention of recurrent problems

Potential risks associated with bursectomy

(a) **Excessive Bleeding-** Excess bleeding during the recovery process or the surgery itself is a potential risk although the risk is usually alleviated by the surgeon's proficiency and cautious observation during the procedure.

(b) **Discomfort and Pain-** Postoperative is usual after a bursectomy, and while it is controlled with pain medications all through the recovery phase, each individual's experience will be distinctive in terms of pain tolerance.

(c) **Formation of blood clot-** Surgery can elevate the risk of blood clot formation, potentially leading to medical complications such as *deep vein thrombosis.* Conservative measures like physical therapy and several medications can help in preventing this type of risk during the recovery process.

(d) **Scarring-** Any surgery carries the risk of noticeable scars at the incision site. Scarring is extremely dependent on the distinctive characteristics of each patient, and will be closely observed on each follow-up consultation or visit.

(e) **Joint weakness/stiffness-** There is a potential risk of a temporary joint weakness/stiffness following a bursectomy procedure and this is common during the early stages of recovery. Physical therapy is important in addressing and reducing this problem. Physical therapy which help patients in regaining strength, range of motion, as well as enhancing the general quality of life is crucial in addressing the reducing these problems.

(f) **Infections-** There is a potential risk of an infection from a bursectomy, although the use of antibiotics during the surgery helps in reducing the possible risk of infection.

Bursitis can likely be improved with treatment, although if bursitis becomes chronic, it may be as a result of:

- *Inappropriate diagnosis and inappropriate treatment*
- *An underlying health condition that can't be cured.*

Other home remedies for bursitis may include:

(a) Resting and avoiding overusing the affected area

(b) Applying ice to decrease swelling for the first 2 days (48 hours) after symptoms occur

(c) Applying dry or moist heat, such as *making use of a heating pad or taking a warm bath.*

(d) Cushioning the knees if you sleep on your side by positioning a small pillow between your legs.

(e) Taking an *over-the-counter* medication, such as **ibuprofen or naproxen sodium** to ease pain and decrease inflammation.

CONCLUSION

Bursitis is an inflammation (irritation) of the bursae or a throbbing condition that affects the small, fluid-filled sacs referred to as **Bursae.** The Bursae which are more than 150 in the human body are fluid-filled sacs located around your joints that surrounds, lubricates, or shields the areas where tendons, skin, and muscle tissues meet bones. Inflamed bursae which results into pain and discomfort in the affected location limit the ways an individual can move their joints. Injury, excessive-use, or inflammation from gout or an autoimmune condition such as *rheumatoid arthritis* may result into bursitis.

THE END.

www.ingramcontent.com/pod-product-compliance
Lightning Source LLC
Chambersburg PA
CBHW071553260726
48653CB00008BA/3076